RSI

Edward C Huskisson

Consultant Physician and Rheumatologist

St Bartholomew's Hospital and

King Edward VII Hospital for Officers, London

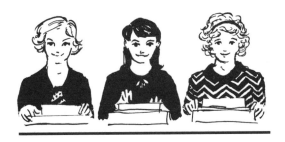

Illustrated by Dodie Masterman

Foreword by Richard Pearson

Charterhouse Conference and
Communication Company Limited

First Edition 1992

ISBN 0-9519807-0-X

Published by Charterhouse Conference and Communications Limited, 35 Cloth Fair, London EC1A 7JQ. Tel: 071-606 2435.

Designed and typeset by Karen Peskett Ltd and printed by Wizard Printing.

British Library Cataloguing-in-Publication Data. A catalogue record for this book is available from the British Library.

About the Author

Ted Huskisson is Consultant Physician and Rheumatologist, Senior Lecturer in Medicine and Head of the Rheumatology Department at St Bartholomew's Hospital London. He is also a member of the staff of King Edward VII Hospital for Officers and has a busy private practice in Queen Anne Street.

Dr Huskisson graduated in 1964 from the Westminster Hospital, London and moved to St Bartholomew's as Senior Registrar in 1970; shortly after this he became Consultant to the Rheumatology Department. He is a member of the British Society for Rheumatology, served on the Education Committee of the Arthritis and Rheumatism Council and was Heberden Roundsman in 1987.

Dr Huskisson is a world authority and is renowned for his lectures on various aspects of rheumatic diseases. He has written over 300 papers on the subject and is Editor of the European Journal of Rheumatology and Inflammation. He has already written his first book "All the Arthropathies" which is now in its 4th edition, and "Repetitive Strain Injury – the Keyboard Disease" is the first in a series of medical books for the Charterhouse Health Series.

He has taken a particular interest in RSI, having travelled to Australia on several occasions to witness the phenomenon at first hand and has established an RSI clinic in the rheumatology department at St Bartholomew's.

I wish to thank the many people who helped in various ways with this book. My special thanks must go to Abigail Gill whose editorial assistance ensured the success of the project.

Contents

Foreword

"REPETITIVE STRAIN SYNDROME", or less controversially "work-related upper limb disorder" is becoming an increasing area of interest. But controversy surrounds even the nomenclature, and the use of the term RSI is deplored by various influential bodies. The vague description of symptoms, difficulty in localising physical signs and lack of a clearly defined pathological basis for the conditions, all make it the subject of argument and speculation. The role of treatment, in particular the use by some physiotherapists of adverse mechanical tension techniques, and the time course of recovery make management of this condition the subject of debate. To this may be added the psychological disturbance suffered by many patients. The need to liaise with co-professionals, including counsellors, physiotherapists and personnel officers and the need to provide frequent reports, compound the reluctance of some doctors to involve themselves in the care of such patients.

Management of patients with repetition injuries requires not only knowledge of the medical aspects of the condition and its subtle complications, but also familiarity with various aspects of ergonomics, physiotherapy, health and safety advice, employment law and industrial psychology in order to provide the best possible care. All those involved in the care of patients need to continually update their knowledge of this rapidly expanding subject and will then find it satisfying as well as challenging. The problem of workplace upper limb disorder is likely to increase; not only in the number of sufferers but also in its impact on the work place, as the need for data-handling increases throughout the world.

Richard Pearson

RSI Clinic

Department of Rheumatology

St Bartholomew's Hospital

Introduction

This book is dedicated to the losers in the RSI story, the patients who suffered pain, loss of work, loss of earnings, and their employers who had to manage without them, pay them off or even compensate them. It is the story of a medical disaster which has come about because of changes in technology, particularly the arrival of fast keyboards and the organisation of work practises so that employees are required to do one job all day. Keyboard workers brought the disease to prominence because there are so many of them. Once upon a time, secretaries typed and filed and answered the telephone. In the drive for efficiency in the last decade or two, it was seen as expedient to have a worker using a keyboard all day. But it was not a good idea. The epidemic was amplified by a type of mass hysteria, encouraged by doctors, lawyers, women's magazines and feminist organisations (for most victims are women) and trade unions, the winners in the story, all of whom saw benefits of various kinds.

RSI is a painful condition usually affecting the hands and forearms. It is, as the name implies, a consequence of repetitive muscular contraction, not necessarily but usually at work. RSI is not new - the name is new but the condition has existed since work began. It wasn't a big problem until an epidemic in Australia brought it to prominence. The epidemic began at the beginning and ended at the end of the 1980's. Towards the end of the eighties it started in the UK and is now an enormous problem. We are fortunate to be able to examine recorded experience of the Australian epidemic, to learn from mistakes which were made in handling a difficult situation and to react sensibly to the threat of our own epidemic.

Well before the end of the 1990's, RSI will be as boring as it has become in Australia. Work practises will have changed. Employers and employees will be aware of the potential problem and doctors and lawyers will be more sensible in dealing with it. But in the meantime many thousands of victims will suffer from a catastrophe which is both predictable and preventable.

CHAPTER 1

The Facts – In A Nutshell

There is considerable argument about many aspects of RSI, whether it is a real disease, whether it exists at all, whether it is organic or psychogenic and so on. But there are a series of facts which stand out as central to the RSI story and I shall recite them now.

What is RSI?

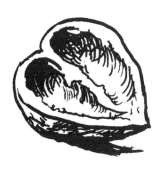

If you do manual work for a few hours without stopping and if you do the same with any muscle group, you will start to ache. This is normal and presumably physiological, a warning that a spell of rest would be a good idea. The development of this aching will depend upon many factors including your physical fitness, your accustomednesss to the task, stress (the wife yelling from the kitchen, " When are you coming to help with the washing up?" etc etc), the weather, the force required, equipment used (that broken screwdriver wasn't such a good plan), your position (you should have borrowed Uncle Jack's ladder) and your work rate ("If you don't get it finished tonight, you'll have to get your own dinner"). When you rest (and with the help of a large gin and tonic) the aching goes.

If you are sitting in a room full of people doing the same thing and those around you start to complain of pain which seems to be caused by the very same thing that you are doing, there is a much greater chance that you will also develop pain than if you were in a room of uncomplaining colleagues. It may be said the same is true of boats. If anyone gets out a brown paper bag, even if its just his sandwiches, everyone feels sick. It's a universal experience.

If you continue to carry out the manual or other activity which caused the pain, the pain will become more severe and more persistent. This usually happens over weeks and months rather than hours or days. Eventually, if you persist with the activity which caused the pain, the pain will fail to resolve even with

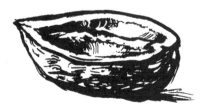

rest. The more severe the pain, and the more persistent, when you eventually decide to quit, the longer will your recovery take. This is called RSI.

Why RSI?

RSI stands for Repetition (or repetitive) Strain Injury; I prefer Repetitive Strain Syndrome but many people have tried to change the name of the condition and have failed, as I shall fail. RSI it is and RSI it will be. A list of alternative names is given in the following table:

Alternative Names for RSI

1. Repetition (or repetitive) Strain Injury or Syndrome (RSI)

2. Occupational Overuse Syndrome (OOS)

3. Overuse Syndrome

4. Muscle Overuse Syndrome

5. Occupational Cervico-brachial Disorder (OCD)

6. Cumulative Trauma Disorder (CTD)

7. Regional Pain Syndrome

8. Localised Fibrositis or Fibromyalgia Syndrome

9. Chronic Upper Limb Pain Syndrome

10. Occupational Neuralgia, cramp, palsy or neurosis (see Chapter 2)

11. Work- related Upper Limb Disorder

12. Refractory Cervico-Brachial Pain (RCBP)

13. Static Stress Syndrome

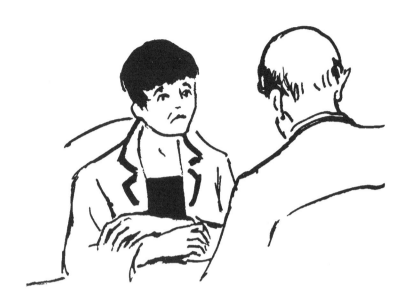

An Unsatisfactory Consultation

Patient: *I have a pain in my arm*

Doctor: *You have "Arm Pain Syndrome"*

Patient: *...(thinks)... Silly old fool. I should have gone to a specialist*

The number of alternatives reflects the confusion about the condition although within these titles, each carefully thought out and proposed by an optimist hoping for acceptance of his proposition, are the essential features of RSI. It is repetition which causes overuse, although whether it is an injury is disputed, which led the Australians to propose alternatives. Strain is a non-medical word with no exact medical meaning but there is no doubt that it is now enshrined in the literature

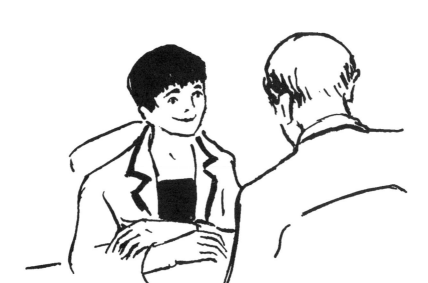

A Satisfactory Consultation

Patient: *I have a pain in my arm*

Doctor: *You have "R S I"*

Patient: *Oh yes, Gladys at work has that*

---

on this subject. RSI sounds nice - OOS doesn't (see previous table). But there is repetition, there is overuse, a cumulative trauma and it is usually but not always occupational. The striking failure of treatment in RSI led to the term "Refractory" and it usually but not always affects the upper limb, hence cervico-brachial - the neck and arm. Recognising that nothing is known of the nature or cause of the condition, some have proposed entirely meaningless terms like Regional Pain Syndrome.

Why Bother with a Diagnosis?

A diagnosis is very important. It enables doctors to communicate with each other and with patients. It may not matter if the names themselves fail to describe the disease and there are so many diseases for which the causes are unknown, that confusion is inevitable. We all accept the name "Polymyalgia Rheumatica" for a disease which doesn't affect muscles although patients often think it does. The diagnosis must however convey to the patient that the doctor knows the cause of the problem, has categorised it and can therefore draw upon the body of medical knowledge which exists to suggest treatment and to advise about outcome.

What RSI is NOT!

It is equally important to talk about what is not RSI and three types of soft tissue rheumatism are particularly important in this respect.

RSI IS NOT	● **Tennis Elbow**
● **Tennis Elbow**	● **Tenosynovitis**
● **Tenosynovitis**	● **Carpal Tunnel Syndrome**
● **Carpal Tunnel Syndrome**	**IS NOT RSI**

Tennis Elbow is an inflammation of the attachment of the forearm muscles to the bony prominence on the outer aspect of the elbow. The junction of the muscle tendon and bone is called an enthesis and inflammation of this specialised biological "glue" is an enthesitis. It is caused by abnormal muscular contraction, sometimes a minor injury or unusual mechanical circumstances such as a change of tennis racquet. A few cases arise from tennis, most from stresses and strains at home (housewives stirring pudding, or their husbands doing DIY at the weekend) or at work; some just appear for no obvious reason. Tennis elbows are very common in people doing repetitive manual work. Most tennis elbows (perhaps 75%) respond to a steroid injection into the tender area. Most (perhaps 98%) resolve spontaneously after anything up to two years regardless of treatment. In RSI, there is often a "tennis elbow", tenderness at the appropriate site but the response to injection and the outcome are quite different - injection is either ineffective or gives very transient relief and the condition may take a lot more than two years to resolve.

Tenosynovitis is an inflammation of tendon sheaths usually produced by some unusual activity. When the people of East London left the city in the autumn to pick hops, the unaccustomed forearm activity lead to a tenosynovitis which was called "Hoppers Gout". The forearm was often swollen and tender and a hand placed on the affected tendon sheath during movement detected a leathery grating sensation called crepitus. Tenosynovitis can occur in any of the

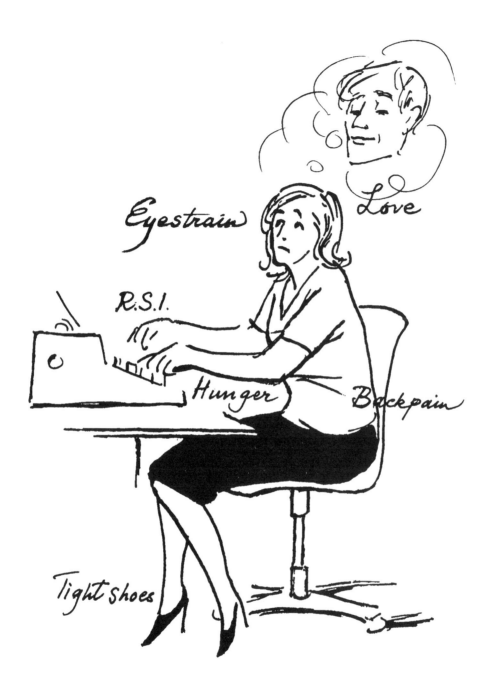

Work is painful

tendon sheaths of the hand and arm and not surprisingly, it is common in people with manual occupations. The swelling, localised tenderness and crepitus are not features of RSI in which symptoms are typically diffuse. Steroid injections are spectacularly effective in tenosynovitis but not in RSI.

Carpal Tunnel Syndrome is a nerve compression at the wrist. The median nerve, which supplies sensation to most of the hand, passes through a tunnel with the blood vessels and tendons which also serve the hand. If the tendons swell or the wrist joint swells as in arthritis or the soft tissues enlarge as in pregnancy, the space reserved for the nerve is compromised. When this happens, the patient wakes at night with pins and needles in the hand and often with pain in the arm and hand. Electrical conduction in the nerve can be measured and is usually abnormal, demonstrating a slowing of the impulse at the level of the wrist. Injection of steroid into the tunnel is spectacularly successful in relieving the symptoms and when it isn't, a minor operation is required to decompress the nerve. Patients with RSI sometimes have symptoms which sound like carpal tunnel syndrome but electrical tests are usually normal, and injecting the carpal tunnel doesn't work; nor does surgical decompression.

So...What is RSI?

Definition

RSI is a condition, usually occupational, characterised by pain which arises in a particular area, usually the hand and forearm, as a result of repetitive muscle activity responding at first to rest but not to treatments appropriate to other types of soft tissue rheumatism such as tenosynovitis, tennis elbow or carpal tunnel syndrome.

When does normal post-exercise or after-work pain become RSI? Perhaps when it starts to interfere with work or other activities; perhaps when it starts to get worse and spreads to other areas, when the vicious cycle of reflexes is set in motion.

CHAPTER 2

A History Lesson

The earliest civilisations must surely have had cases of RSI even though they called it something else. Leather beaters in Ancient Egypt are thought to have been affected but Bernadino Ramazzini in his book on Diseases of Workers, published in 1713, is credited with the first description. He was Professor of Medicine in Modena and then in Padua and is one of the fathers and founders of Occupational Medicine. He wrote that "incessant driving of the pen over paper causes intense fatigue of the hand and the whole arm because of the continuous and almost tonic strain of the muscles and tendons, which in the course of time, results in failure of power in the right hand". Aware of the involvement of the nervous system as a whole, he noted that "what tortures these workers most acutely is the intense and incessant application of the mind, for in work such as this the whole brain, its nerves and fibres, must be constantly on the stretch; hence ensues loss of tonus". Ramazzini described two of the main manifestations of RSI, pain and weakness. English physicians at the end of the 19th Century struggled with the classification of this and other problems which arose from repetitive work and also with the question of causation. Just as Australians argued in their epidemic, some favouring an organic injury and others a psychological origin, English and European physicians at the turn of the century were divided about the cause of these occupational disorders. They were called "occupational neuroses", a term which at the time meant a disorder of the nervous system rather than a psychological abnormality, the current meaning. Psychological abnormalities were however noted by many authors.

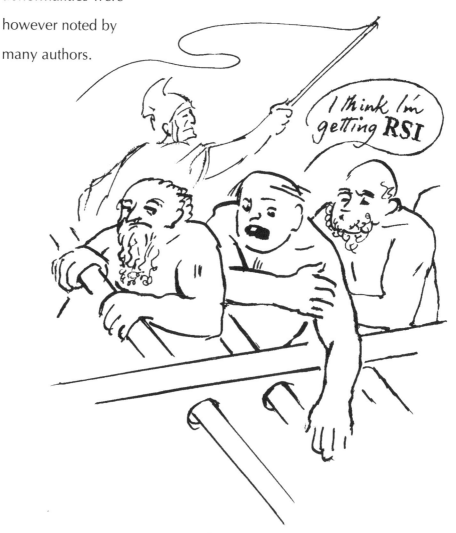

RSI is not a new disease

William Gowers, a famed London neurologist who worked at University College Hospital and the National Hospital for the Paralysed and Epileptic, now the National Hospital for Nervous Diseases, noted in his text book on Diseases Of The Nervous System published in 1892 that these conditions occurred in those of nervous temperament, irritable, sensitive, bearing overwork and anxiety badly. Three main manifestations of these occupational neuroses were identified; pain, weakness or fatigue and cramp. They account for considerable confusion in the literature with similar cases described as occupational neuroses, neuralgias, palsies and cramps. There are many papers on the problems of individual occupations or "craft palsies" including writer's cramp but it is now clear that these are all manifestations of the same basic mechanism; patients with RSI have various combinations of pain, fatigue and cramp.

Writing seems to have been the main cause of RSI in the last century. Writers were called scriveners and the disease was called "Scriveners Palsy". It was well described by Samuel Solly, a physician at St Thomas' Hospital in 1864. He wrote of severe and persistent arm pain accompanied by other sensory symptoms which affected men whose occupations demanded that they write incessantly. The pain was burning or aching in character and was accompanied by a feeling of cold and fatigue and numbness in the fingers. Some patients had cramps and it was either this or pain and fatigue which eventually caused them to stop writing. It was often necessary for these patients to stop working. Solly thought that overwork caused damage to a nerve centre in the spinal cord or the brain.

The variety of terms used in the 19th Century illustrates the spectrum of symptoms which arises from repetitive manual work.

The Occupational Neuroses		
Sensory Symptoms	**Motor Symptoms**	
Pain	Fatigue	Cramp
"Occupational Neuralgia"	"Occupational Palsy"	"Occupational Cramp"

William Gowers reported in 1877 in the Medical Times and Gazette on two cases of writer's cramp. One man had written for ten hours a day over 20 years; the other had done a very moderate amount of daily writing. The former recovered, the latter didn't. Gowers used this experience to point out that there were two aspects to the cause, the stimulus and a predisposition. The smaller the stimulus required to produce writer's cramp, the greater must be the predisposition, he argued. As to treatment, his major recommendation was absolute rest and he advised right-handed patients to learn to write with their left hand which can be done by " a man of average industry and perseverance in the course of a few weeks"!

But it was a friend of William Gowers, George Poore, also a physician at University College Hospital who was the man to see about RSI at the end of the last century. He collected seventy five cases of writer's cramp and impaired writing power which he reported in 1878; by 1887, he had one hundred and sixty eight, a poor rate of progress by today's standards. In most, fatigue prevented writing, but in some there were cramps and in some there was pain. He noted many of the features which have been redescribed recently including tenderness, particularly found along the course of nerves and hyperaesthesia (excessive sensitivity). Some of his patients were pianists and Sir John Russel Reynolds, in his textbook of 1872, noted that the same condition could occur in artists, musicians, seamstresses, smiths and milkmaids.

Physicians in other parts of the world were equally aware of the problem and wrote about it. Professor Austin Flint, a New York physician who is immortalised in the heart murmur that bears his name, wrote about writer's cramp in his textbook and the Boston neurologist W E Paul reviewed two hundred cases of Occupational Neurosis in 1911. Charles Dana, Professor of Neurology at Cornell University collected a hundred cases in 1920; they were writers, telegraphers transmitting the Morse code, stenographers, typists, musicians, pressers, ironers or tailors. It has been going on for a long time.

CHAPTER 3

Why Does It Happen?

Mechanisms and Explanations

Muscles

Prolonged or excessive use of muscles causes injury. It is a universal experience. Using or overusing a particular muscle group eventually

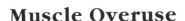

Muscle Overuse

causes pain and there is experimental evidence to support the view that this is an injury. Histological changes are seen in overused muscle and there is a release of muscle enzymes and myoglobin, the muscle protein, into the circulation. Running a marathon is a simple way of damaging muscles and demonstrating these phenomena. The severity of the injury is strictly proportional to the intensity and duration of the activity and these changes are followed by recovery. Muscle pain in these circumstances is probably due to the accumulation of metabolites like lactic acid which are simply removed in the recovery phase.

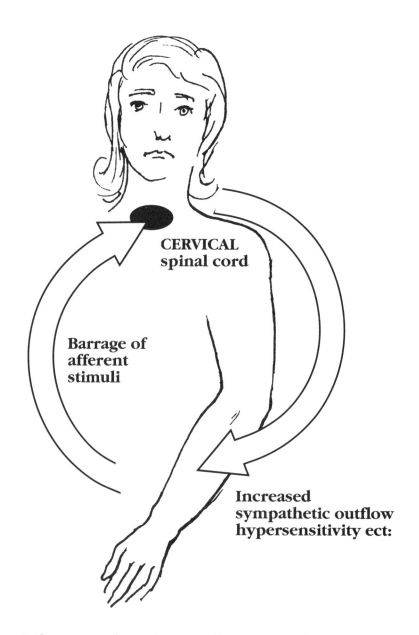

The Mechanism of RSI – First Stage

A barrage of impulses from injured muscle activates the reflex arc and causes increased output from the cervical spinal cord sympathetic nervous system, in turn causing hypersensitivity, changes in colour and temperature etc etc.

The Spinal Cord

It is immediately obvious that this simple mechanism does not explain the phenomenon of RSI. There is evidence of involvement of the spinal cord and it seems likely that a barrage of sensory input leads to an increased output, the activation of a reflex arc. Evidence for spinal cord involvement includes increased sympathetic nervous outflow producing changes in colour, temperature and sweating. The pain in RSI has a "neural" quality, like neuralgia, burning and aching. The McGill pain questionnaire confirms this conclusion. There are abnormalities of sensation such as reduced two point discrimination, the ability to distinguish two pin pricks applied close together. There is hyperalgesia, an abnormal and excessive pain in response to simple mechanical stimulation, as well as hyperaesthesia. Finally it is characteristic that the pain in RSI starts in one area but spreads to others and this is likely to be due to changes within the nervous system.

The Central Nervous System

In RSI, stimulus and response are not related. The same amount of work does not always cause the same problem and it is clear that things happening in the central part of the nervous system, the brain, can influence the development and perception of pain.

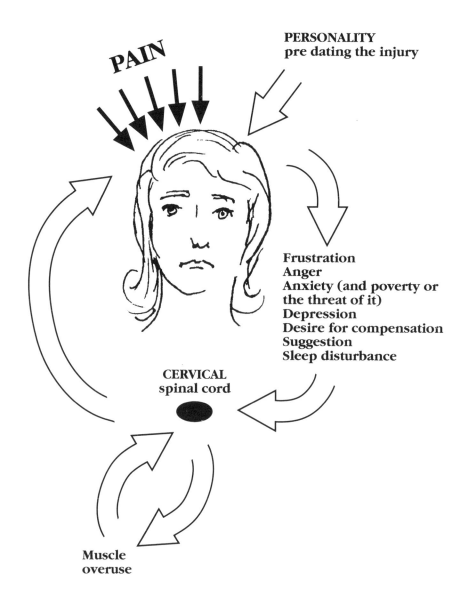

PAIN

PERSONALITY
pre dating the injury

Frustration
Anger
Anxiety (and poverty or
the threat of it)
Depression
Desire for compensation
Suggestion
Sleep disturbance

CERVICAL
spinal cord

Muscle
overuse

The Mechanism of RSI – Second Stage

The reflex arc is influenced by changes in the brain; firstly by the patients personality and secondly by the effects of the pain itself including frustration and anger at the pain and worry about the consequences.

The brain is heavily involved in the experience of pain. To support this view, it is usual to quote soldiers in battle, or football players who feel the pain of their injuries only when the battle is over or the final whistle blown. A handy explanation for this is that the brain acts on the spinal cord to close a gate mechanism which prevents pain impulses from reaching the brain, where the sensation of pain arises. The converse is also true. Changes in the brain can cause the gate to open, lowering the threshold for pain or even allowing the pain to be perceived in the absence of an appropriate physical stimulus. Pain is a common complaint in patients with psychiatric conditions like depression.

Two types of central influence act on the development and perception of pain in RSI. The patient's personality, established long before the development of the condition, may predispose to it. The same is true of some other types of functional muscle disease including fibromyalgia and irritable bowel syndrome. The pain of RSI and other problems associated with the condition may aggravate and reinforce the symptoms. It is not surprising that some sufferers become frustrated and angry at their predicament, especially if their treatment at work or by the medical profession is unsympathetic. Their livelihood is threatened; it is not surprising that anxiety and depression may follow. It is hard to escape the conclusion that compensation has a role to play in this sort of condition. At the very least, the quest for compensation delays recovery. Suggestion or mass hysteria seems to be enormously important in the RSI story and is

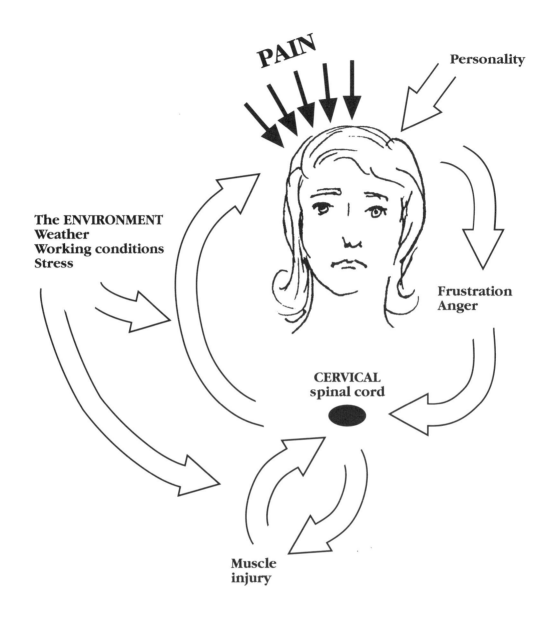

The Mechanism of RSI – Third Stage

The whole complex interaction of injury, reflex arcs, personality, anxiety and other changes resulting from pain are influenced by the environment, the weather, the condition of adjacent workers and working conditions including stress.

discussed in greater detail in chapter 4 and chapter 7. Pain in RSI interferes with sleep and this causes a vicious cycle of muscle spasm and further sleep disturbance. There is an intimate relationship between sleep and muscle, well exemplified by fibromyalgia. Healthy individuals deprived of delta sleep, the deep refreshing part of the cycle develop muscular pain and stiffness which in turn, makes their beds uncomfortable and sleep more difficult. This vicious cycle is part of the fibromyalgia syndrome and it can also occur in RSI.

The Environment

There is one more important aspect of the mechanism of RSI, the environment. Conditions of work are particularly important and RSI is more likely when there is stress at work, monotony and boredom, lack of satisfaction and pressure to achieve targets. It is much more likely to occur when work is carried out in confined spaces with poor lighting and atmosphere. The weather influences the development of a variety of rheumatic problems including fibromyalgia and other types of soft tissue rheumatism.

Alternative Theories

Reference has already been made to the argument about the relative importance of psychological factors and disordered functioning of the nervous system. I argue that both are involved and that the relative importance of physical, psychological and environmental factors varies from case to case but it is worth emphasising that RSI is a functional disorder of muscles and of the nervous system. No consistent structural abnormality has been demonstrated.

Referred pain from the neck has been suggested as an alternative theory and there is no doubt that pressure on nerve roots by a disc prolapse for example, can cause pain and tingling in the hand. It is however difficult to understand why the neck should be the initiating factor in a disease which nearly always starts in the hand. The neck is usually normal in cases of RSI and no evidence of nerve root compression has been forthcoming.

Abnormal mechanical tension in nerves as a result of muscle dysfunction is another theory and the basis for stretching exercises used by physiotherapists. If the problem were simply due to pressure on peripheral nerves, one would expect to see abnormalities of nerve conduction and in cases with symptoms of carpal tunnel syndrome, one would expect decompression to be effective - but it isn't. The problem is more complex.

CHAPTER 4

The Australian Epidemic – and Experience Elsewhere

The epidemic of RSI in Australia is documented in the following diagram which is based partly on recording of cases. Unfortunately the system of reporting was changed in 1987, part of the campaign to "close down RSI" and comparable figures were no longer available. The picture has therefore been completed with a bit of imagination. It must be close to the truth! The UK epidemic is about ten years behind.

The epidemic started in Australia in the early 1980's and gathered momentum over the course of a few years.

Why Did It Begin?

The major factor in starting the epidemic must surely have been the new technology, the introduction of fast keyboards. But these were introduced all over the world; why did it happen in Australia and why has it happened ten years later in the UK? Many other

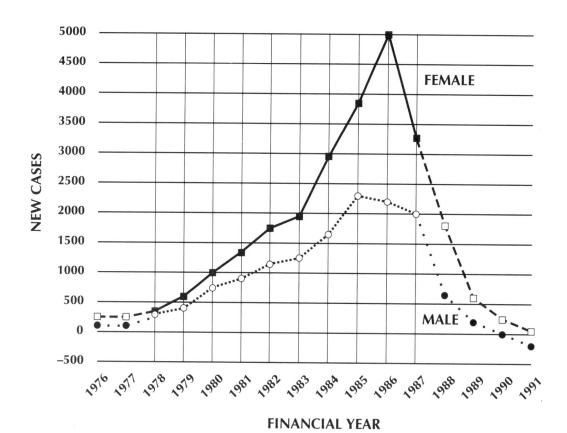

The rise and fall of RSI in Australia

The data for years, 1978 to 1987 are real; the rest is extrapolation.

factors have been identified which explain the "spread" of the disease in Australia. And spread is not an inappropriate term when one considers the striking differences between workers at different sites. For example 25% of a group of telephonists in Sydney developed RSI compared to only 4% of a group of workers doing exactly the same job with exactly the same equipment in Melbourne. It is impossible to escape the conclusion that the disease spreads in the workplace and clusters of cases have been seen wherever RSI appears. Some local epidemics were characterised mainly by pain while in others muscle spasm was the dominant feature. And why, it has been asked, did so many people get RSI in the early 1980's when some offices were rendered non-functional and others were almost unaffected?

RSI in Australia has been described as a major medical blunder. Bell, writing in 1989 and reviewing events calls it "an iatrogenic epidemic of simulated injury". Doctors were quick to diagnose RSI and to provide the necessary certification. They encouraged patients to take on the sick role. Compensation followed without too much difficulty and workers were able to recover their usual wages. Ergonomists piled in to get their share of the action and the advice given to keyboard workers, although well motivated and entirely sensible, must have increased the number of complainers. Pain is normal at the end of the working day, and warning workers to stop working at the first sign of pain must increase their awareness of the problem.

The majority of workers affected by RSI were female - most keyboard workers are female -and feminist groups became involved. Trade unions came to support their members in their quest for compensation. Wild ideas were circulated; it was suggested for example that outmoded Japanese-made keyboards had been dumped on the Australian market or that the rays emitted from VDU screens were the cause of the trouble. An atmosphere of hostility was generated against employers.

It is argued that the use of the term "injury" also promoted the epidemic. If people have been injured they have been impaired and must be compensated. They must seek redress against those who injured them. It is acceptable to have been injured; it is worthy of sympathy. RSI was a socially acceptable disease.

Why Did It End?

There was a turning point in the Australian epidemic. It occurred at the beginning of the second half of the decade and it lead to the virtual disappearance of RSI in Australia. There is no doubt that working practises had changed. Employers made sure that employees were not at risk from this disease; an expensive lesson had been learned. But many other things happened. Doctors certainly saw that their activities were perpetuating the problem and in 1986, the Royal Australasian College of Physicians published an extraordinary statement making several points. First, it stated that there was no scientific evidence that the symptoms of

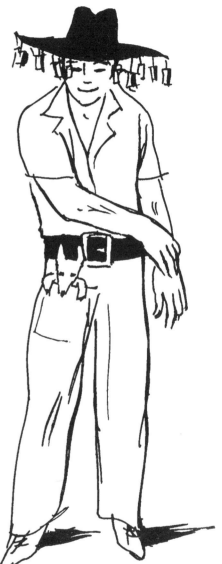

"Kangaroo paw"

RSI were attributable to work practises. It contrasted RSI with common workplace injuries such as tenosynovitis in which there is well established pathology, nomenclature and treatment. Second it disputed the presence of injury: patients..."perceive themselves as being injured. This is not so". Third, it criticised the media for misuse of information, and unions, support groups and colleagues of patients who though acting in the best interests of the patients, through naivety, fuelled the flames and amplified the symptoms. The disease was seen as psychosomatic although the vast majority of patients was acknowledged to have genuine symptoms. The Royal Australasian College of Physicians concluded that the availability of compensation and legal action to obtain compensation had served the patients very poorly.

Some companies tried to screen employees prior to employment with a view to detecting and rejecting RSI prone individuals. Thus a clothing company surveyed twelve hundred employees, 90% of whom were female, claiming that small fat women were prone to the disease and advising against their employment. This was reported in a journal called WRIST, the Womens Repetition Injury Support Team, no doubt one of the organisations held responsible for perpetuating the problem.

The media joined in the fun and articles appeared in newspapers on the same theme. The disease was given the name "kangaroo paw", a term of derision. In 1987 a journalist got himself employed in a clothing factory, faked the symptoms of RSI, was readily diagnosed and certified by a doctor and received $4000 Australian dollars in compensation from the government. This story was the subject of a television programme and at the time there was widespread anti-RSI publicity. RSI had become socially unacceptable.

The Cost of RSI

The cost must have been massive. In the five years up to 1987, covering the peak of the epidemic, Telecom Australia is said to have lost $15 million Australian dollars (about £6.5 million pounds sterling) because of RSI. The estimated cost of the whole epidemic to Australian industry in the years up to 1989 was half a billion Australian dollars (about £220 million sterling) - expensive!

The cost in human terms was also massive and many will continue to suffer and be disadvantaged for many years to come.

The Ballad of RSI

In 1986, Rick Travers, a Rheumatologist from Melbourne, wrote a poem about RSI. It captures the spirit of the time and is reproduced with the kind permission of the author.

Towards A Ballad Of RSI

"Some to the fascination of a name
surrender judgement hoodwinked"

William Cowper

Railway Spine was the first to come
Then Shell-Shock during World War 1
Then backs, then Whiplash (a pain in the bum!)
And now we have RSI.

Beware if e'er the forearm aches:
A few hours' work is all it takes.
To save your arm, apply the brakes -
Or be crippled by RSI.

O.T.'s will splint you by night and by day
And check that the TENS machine's working OK.
Ergonomists whip chair and keyboard away
Which caused your RSI.

Caring Psychologists help you relax.
Physios' waves heat up muscles or backs,
While it's needles and diets (Good grief!) from the Quacks
It's an industry, RSI.

The carpal tunnel's been decompressed
But the pain continues - well, I'm blessed!
You'll need another year of rest -
That's the thing about RSI.

The Specialist says that the pain isn't real -
Well, how would he know how you feel?
Your GP will say, if you give him the spiel,
That you're unfit, with RSI.

The lawyer says "This injury
should yield a lump sum (and my fee)
within a year ... two ... or three -
It's a gold-mine this RSI.

Maybe that's so - you might do alright
But it's several years off, and a hard bloody fight
Each round of which adds to the sufferer's plight -
The winner is RSI.

RSI in the USA

Much less is known of RSI in the USA. Figures however suggest that it is common and increasing. Thus in 1988, 48% of the 24,000 workplace illnesses in private business were due to cumulative trauma disorders, the accepted name for RSI in the USA - this compares with only 18% in 1981. The National Institute for Occupational Safety and Health estimated in 1991 that 5 million Americans suffered from RSI and that 50% of the workforce would be at risk by the year 2000. By this time, it was thought that 75 % of all jobs would involve the use of computers. RSI has never achieved the same publicity in the USA as it did in Australia, perhaps because of deliberate policy.

Two notable epidemics have been reported. One occurred in telephonists, specifically those dealing with directory enquiries. The same disparity was noted between people doing the same work in different states, as was noted in Australia. Patients who did particularly badly and were least likely to recover, were those involved in medical treatment outside their workplace, those treated surgically and those involved in litigation. The direct cost of compensation paid to workers by the telephone company was $1.5 million US dollars (£850,000 Sterling). Ergonomists played a big part in the affair and there were arguments, some conducted in the law courts, about the role of different types of keyboards. However changes in the keyboard did not lead to a drop in the number of cases and no ergonomic variable could be discerned which would account for the variation in the number of cases occurring at the different sites.

Another epidemic occurred in postal workers following the introduction of keyboards in place of manual letter sorting in the early 1960's, cases finally reaching the courts some twenty years later. It was said that 50% of operators, who were required to enter one post code every second, reported pain in their hand, arms, neck and shoulders. The post office refused to accept that their machines were responsible and contested all claims.

There is said to be a class action underway on behalf of a group of children alleging damage from the use of computer games, a mini epidemic! There are other clusters of cases, including 17% of journalists at the Los Angeles Times, which like the Financial Times in London, seems to have been particularly affected.

RSI in the Third World

There is an enormous potential for the RSI problem in third world countries because of the use of offshore data entry sites. The cost of entering computer data in the Philippines or the Caribbean may be 10% of the cost of doing the same work in the USA. The data can be transmitted to or from the site by telephone and it is therefore an attractive proposition. The work is often paid at least in part on the basis of productivity or with bonuses, making a big incentive to keyboard workers to work for long hours without breaks. Reliable data on the prevalence of RSI are unlikely to be available but the problem undoubtedly exists.

CHAPTER 5

Occupations At Risk

Anyone can get RSI. The following are particularly at risk:

In general

Keyboard Workers   **Process Workers**

Assembly Workers   **Packers**

Machine Operators

In particular

- **Secretaries and typists**
- **Chicken process workers**
- **Telephonists**
- **Mail sorters**
- **Supermarket checkout girls**
- **Journalists**
- **Airline reservation clerks**
- **Metal workers**

- **Fabric sewers and cutters**

- **Clerks**

- **Ledger machinists**

- **Musicians**

- **Dancers**

- **Artists**

- **Cleaners**

- **Potters**

- **Bakers**

- **Dog groomers**

- **Signers for the deaf**

- **Condom lifters**

RSI occurs as a result of leisure activities as well as work. It has been described in players of various games such as Rubik's cube (Cuber's thumb), or computer games (Nintendinitis and Space Invader's wrist). The use of a computer mouse can cause joint pain (mouse joint) or even a trapped nerve (mouse trap)! Slot machine tendinitis was reported after a weekend on the machines and Centenarian Hand Syndrome after a 100th birthday party and lots of hand shaking; it is probably well known to royalty and important persons. Marathon running has received the blame for RSI and it's occurrence in dancers is also a reminder that it can affect the lower

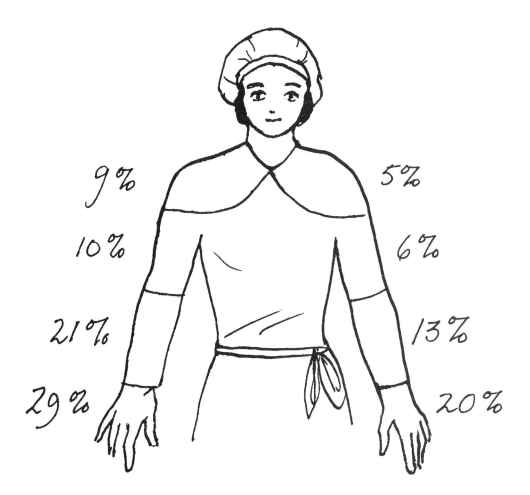

9%   5%

10%   6%

21%   13%

29%   20%

Pain in the arms in chicken process workers

Figures show the percentage of such workers who had regular discomfort in different parts of their right and left arms. The data is taken from a study by Buckle (see appendix 1). For comparison 1–3% of department store or supermarket staff had similar symptoms.

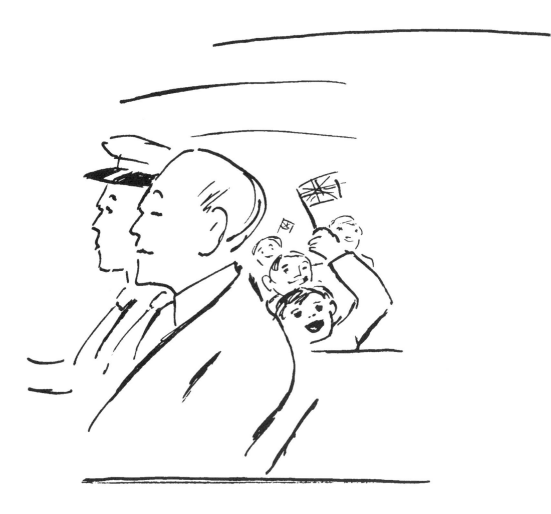

Anyone can

limbs. It is even said to affect the lips of trumpet or trombone players.

Other syndromes which are self-explanatory include television neck

and tennis neck, well known to watchers of the Wimbledon

tournament, dentist's leg, gymnast's; javelin thrower's or judo elbow,

ping pong tenosynovitis, hula hoop syndrome and karate hand.

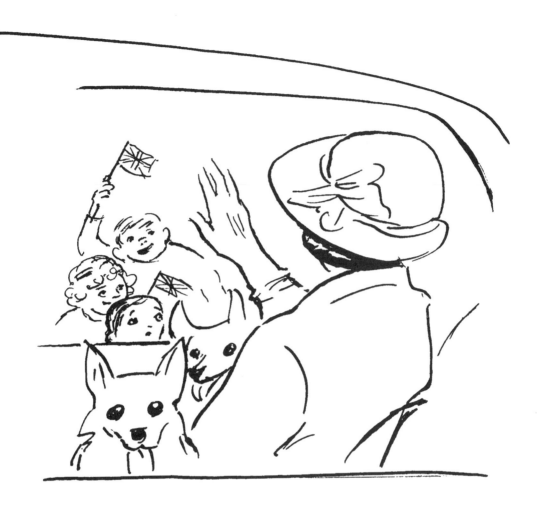

get RSI

We have seen that cramps are one feature of the RSI syndrome and in addition to writer's cramp, many others have been described including ballet-dancer's, bricklayer's, cigarette roller's, dancer's, drummer's, flautist's and most other musical instrument player's, typists and sewer's cramps.

Musicians are at risk from RSI and it is easy to see how enthusiasm could lead to long practice sessions without breaks. An Australian study found 379 cases of painful overuse in the upper limbs of 900 musicians from six symphony orchestras and in the staff and students of nine music schools. In striking contrast to data from other types of worker, the problem was slightly more common in men than in women. All types of musicians were affected but string players were the commonest group and woodwind players were slightly more often affected than keyboard players with the clarinet as the commonest instrument to be blamed.

Workers in the chicken processing business have always been known to suffer particularly from soft tissue rheumatic problems like tennis elbow and they have also suffered greatly from RSI. They are required to carry out multiple manual operations such as trussing, plucking and disembowelment. Not surprisingly the repetitive movements required for these operations cause a lot of upper limb pain.

CHAPTER 6

Symptoms and Signs

Who Gets It?

Women are affected about six times more often than men. The condition occurs mainly between the ages of twenty and fifty with a mean age in the thirties for many of the reported series. For occupations affected, see chapter five.

The Onset

It starts gradually in most cases (about 75%). When it occurs suddenly, there may be a definite episode of trauma or strain which precipitates it. There are a number of important precipitating factors as follows:

- **Change of work**, a move to a new task for example

- **Change of equipment**, a new typewriter for example, and particularly a change from an electrical or mechanical typewriter to a modern high speed keyboard

- **Return to work**, after a holiday or sickness

- **Injury at work**

- **Stress at work**, change of supervisor, new and unsympathetic colleagues

- **Stress and anxiety at home,** marital discord

- **Excessive work load or hours worked**

- **Lack of breaks,** because of pressure of work or desire to go home early

- **Bonuses or incentives**

The Site

It is characteristic that the pain is at first localised, usually to the hands, wrist or forearms. In ninety per cent of cases, one region is affected initially but spread to other areas is common. In twenty five percent of cases, symptoms are felt in both hands and arms at the same time. The shoulder, neck and back may become involved. The dominant limb is much more commonly affected than the non-dominant.

The Symptoms

There is a variable combination of one or more of the following complaints:

- **Pain**, deep and burning with an electrical quality

- **Aggravated by work**. Characteristically the pain occurs first at the end of the day and is relieved overnight. Over the course of weeks and months, if the work is continued, it becomes more severe and more persistent, occurring earlier in the day, not completely relieved by rest at the weekend or on holiday. Eventually it becomes constant and unbearably severe. Some patients are disabled by pain which comes with simple household activities such as brushing their hair or cleaning their teeth.

- **Aggravated by bad weather, cold, damp and stress**. The latter is not surprising - stress, like cold, makes muscles contract and if they are already painful, the pain gets worse

- **Relieved by rest**

- **Pins and needles**, usually in the hands

- **Cramps**

- **Fatigue.** Weakness may interfere with work as much as pain and like cramp, is the dominant feature in some cases

- **A feeling of swelling**

- **Disturbed sleep**. A brief period of morning stiffness occurs in 50% of cases

- **Headaches, irritability and mood changes.**

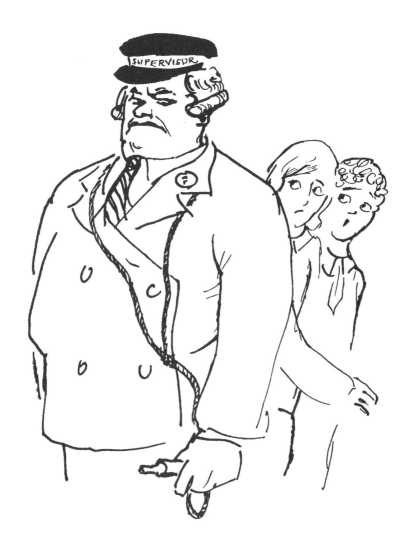

Stress at work

The Signs

It is a characteristic feature of RSI that there are symptoms without signs; the hands feel swollen but aren't, muscles feel weak but aren't wasted or in any other way abnormal. There are no objective physical findings in most cases of RSI. A lack of spontaneous movement is characteristic and the patient may have difficulty with fine finger movements. Rapid fatigue occurs in the performance of set tasks. There may be visible spasms or cramps. The joints feel stiff, meaning that there is a reluctance to move, but the range of movement is full. Tenderness of muscles and tenderness along the lines of nerves may be noted or tenderness over trigger points such as the lateral epicondyle of the elbow. But in many cases, there is absolutely nothing to be found.

Tests

X Rays, blood tests, nerve conduction studies, muscle biopsies and other tests are of no value in RSI except to exclude some other cause for the symptom.

Complications

- **Reflex Sympathetic Dystrophy**. A small proportion of patients with RSI develop an unusual complication called reflex sympathetic dystrophy or algodystrophy. This mysterious condition occurs as a result of fractures about the ankle when it is called Sudeck's Atrophy and is a rare complication of other types of injury, including intracranial and intrathoracic surgery. Sometimes it occurs for no obvious reason; sometimes it is precipitated by some trivial injury. It is characterised by pain and swelling of the affected extremity with vasomotor changes - changes in colour, temperature and sweating. It responds poorly to treatment but usually resolves after a year or two

- **Depression** - not surprising - and even suicide

- **Dystonia and inco-ordination**

CHAPTER 7

Psychological Aspects

The pain ... in strain
... lies mainly in the brain.

Anon (probably Australian!)

It is not surprising that RSI has attracted the attention of psychologists and psychiatrists, trying to claim that it is one of their diseases, psychogenic or at least psychosomatic. Doctors confronted with patients complaining of a set of symptoms try to fit those symptoms into one of their recognised and previously taught frameworks. Thus patients who wake at night with pins and needles in their hands, rub and shake their hands to obtain relief, have carpal tunnel syndrome. When the symptoms don't fit any of the frameworks, it is easy to suspect that the problem is not due to an organic or structural disease. When there are no physical signs and no abnormal tests, the case for psychogenesis is even stronger. But one must be cautious. Angina is a symptom without signs; most patients with carpal tunnel syndrome have symptoms but no signs and even nerve conduction studies are not always abnormal.

Personality

It was fashionable, not so long ago, to think that many chronic diseases including rheumatoid arthritis and ulcerative colitis had their basis in the psychological make-up of the patient. There is a large body of literature on the personality of patients with rheumatoid arthritis who tend to be passive, introverted and submissive. It is of course impossible to predict the development of the disease and therefore impossible to study pre-morbid personality. Most people now believe however that personality changes in these sort of diseases are the result of the disease rather than the cause. It seems less likely that it is the odd personality of patients with ulcerative colitis which makes their bowels open ten times daily; more likely that frequent bowel motions will have an effect on their personality. What effect would the development of painful hands in a manual worker have on their personality with the threat to their livelihood and other problems associated with their condition?

So we don't know whether RSI is a disease which affects people of a certain personality type or whether the disease affects their personalities. There is no doubt that they are anxious people, as noted by Gowers in the last century. Not only were his patients anxious, but he noted that they tended to have family problems, business worry or weighty responsibilities. He thought that this "lowered the tone" of the nervous system. Janet, a French physician of the same period, thought that these occupational problems occurred in "psychasthenics" and that the problem was due to a general lowering of nervous energy. He found patients obsessional, overscrupulous and well behaved. It is worth emphasising that it is not the lazy people on the production line who get RSI; quite the reverse. It is the well-motivated obsessional people who struggle to get all their work done in time!

Mass Hysteria

It is also necessary to discuss, in this context, the concept of mass hysteria and its relevance to RSI. In promoting this view of the Australian epidemic a model was proposed in which there were seven important features:

- **A stressful life** situation generating a conflict about working

- **Everyday aches and pains** or fatigue during the performance of repetitive manual work. There is no doubt that aching is common in keyboard workers at the end of the day, regarded as usual and accepted as part of the deal

- **A strongly held belief** that repetitive movement can injure upper limb tissues

- **Reinforcement** from fellow workers, trade unions, the press and other peer groups

- **Medical diagnosis** and certification from work in the absence of physical signs or supporting of physical evidence of injury or illness

- **A workers compensation scheme**, easy to access

- **A favourable socio-political milieu** for acceptance of RSI as a compensatable condition

Those who favour the theory of mass hysteria blame the spread of RSI in Australia on it and argue that no other theory can explain the time course of the epidemic; people are doing the same jobs today and not getting RSI because several of the essential features described including certification and social acceptability have been removed. No other theory, it is argued, could explain the disparity in incidence between workers at different sites - and for that matter in different countries.

Hysteria, Suggestion and Malingering

The use of the term hysteria is misleading but "mass hysteria" is the usual description of this phenomenon. It should not be confused with conversion hysteria which implies gain of some sort. The vast majority, if not all RSI sufferers, have lost and lost and lost again. RSI is definitely not that sort of hysteria. Nor is it likely to be due to malingering, again because of the absence of gain. There may have been a few scallywags who jumped on the RSI band wagon but they probably jumped off again very quickly. It is much better - financially and emotionally - to be at work. Compensation and the quest for it doesn't make victims happy; in most cases it makes them very unhappy with unrealistic expectations and years of argument and delay. Few RSI sufferers have received more than trivial amounts of compensation; most have received nothing.

Losses in RSI

- **JOB**

- **CAREER**

- **INCOME**

- **INDEPENDENCE**

- **LIFE STYLE**

- **SELF-RESPECT**

- **FUTURE**

The design of the perfect secretary and her workplace

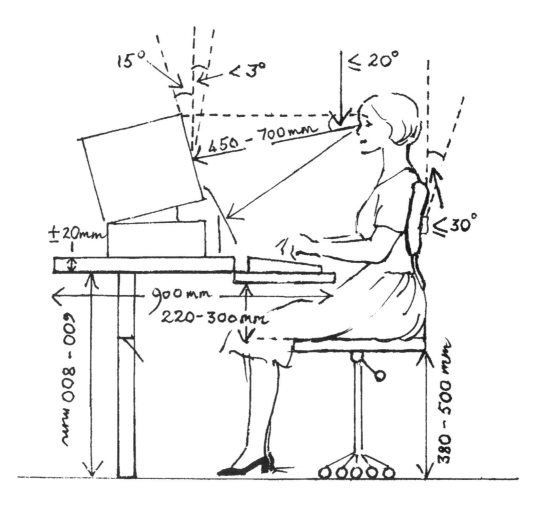

Note that the screen, document holder and keyboard are in the same plane so that she doesn't have to turn her head.

The desk is thin so that there is room for her legs underneath it. Her forearm is horizontal and her wrists are in the neutral position. The chair is covered in permeable fabric.

All the equipment is nice to look at, kind to clothes and safe.

CHAPTER 8

Ergonomics

The Science of the Workplace

For ergonomists, RSI was the answer to the maiden's prayer. They multiplied and measured, taking an inch off the height of the desk and adding a centimetre to the width of the back rest. But did it help? Most commentators have concluded that it didn't. The Royal Australasian College of Physicians opined that the industry developed to correct ergonomic problems in the Australian workplace was excessive. But the legacy of the experience is a large body of information about the organisation of work, the design of the workplace and working tools. The secretarial office will never be the same again.

General Principals

One may divide the factors to be considered as follows:

■ Biomechanical factors

A constrained and inefficient posture is an obvious predisposing factor in RSI. There should be adequate space for each worker, enabling the optimum working position to be adopted for any particular task.

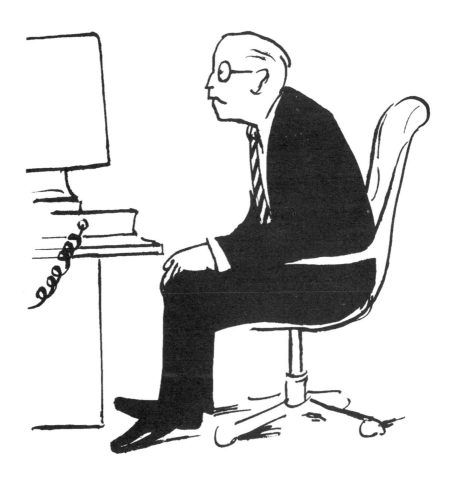

Back problem or eye problem?
Corset or new glasses?

Frequent repetitive movement is the essential biomechanical cause of RSI.

An abnormal or uncomfortable joint position for work procedures may predispose to the development of pain. For keyboard work, hyperextension or hyperflexion of the wrist, or ulnar deviation of the hand at the wrist, can cause pain. Due to incorrect height of chair/desk keeping the wrist bent to its maximum degree quickly causes pain in healthy people - try it! Joints should be in a comfortable position in the middle part of their normal range.

A faulty work station or equipment; broken or badly designed chairs, desks or keyboards obviously cause trouble. There is no convincing evidence that one design of keyboard is any better or worse than any other although there is no doubt that it is modern keyboards which brought about the epidemic of RSI. Some say that the biggest culprit is the word wrap facility which enables the typist to continue indefinitely without the need to operate the carriage return at the end of each line.

Stress; stress causes muscle tension and muscle tension is a major factor in functional muscle diseases like fibromyalga and RSI. Stress may arise from a variety of sources including supervisors, fellow workers and problems at home.

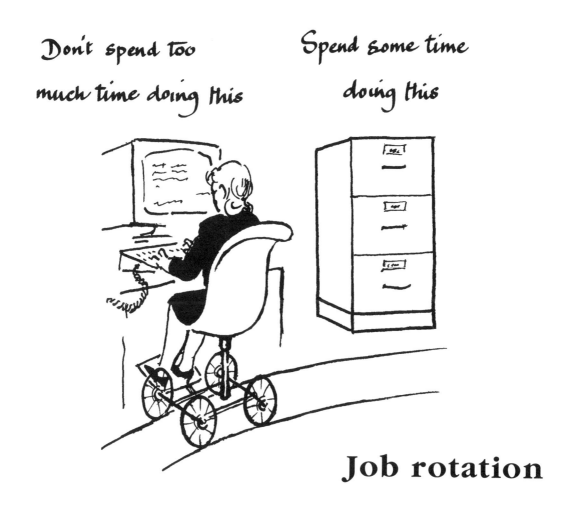

Don't spend too much time doing this

Spend some time doing this

Job rotation

☐ Faulty work organisation

Inadequate rest periods are of great importance. It is madness to operate a keyboard or to carry on any other tasks for long periods without breaks.

Bonus and overtime incentives may cause operators to work for longer hours than is desirable and with shorter breaks.

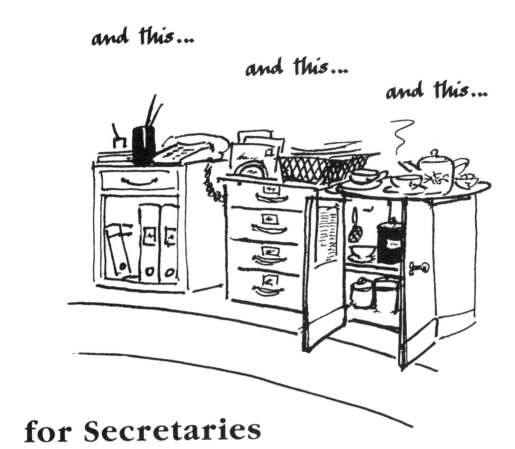

and this...

and this...

and this...

for Secretaries

Lack of training; training should ensure that workers are capable of doing the tasks which they are required to do. A period of training should also provide the opportunity to work slowly up to the required speed of operation.

Failure of supervision.

Bad task design; lack of variety of work or operations badly planned so that they are carried out in awkward positions or inefficiently.

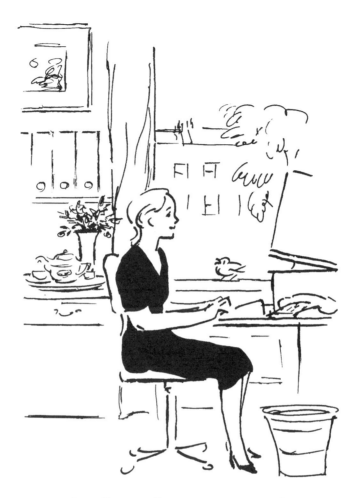

A nice place to work

■ Incompetent personnel

Delayed reporting of problems. Everyone agrees that prevention is
the key to RSI but early reporting is the next best thing. On the other
hand, if manual workers are encouraged to report things that happen
every day like muscular discomfort after work, the development of
epidemics may be encouraged. In steering a middle course between

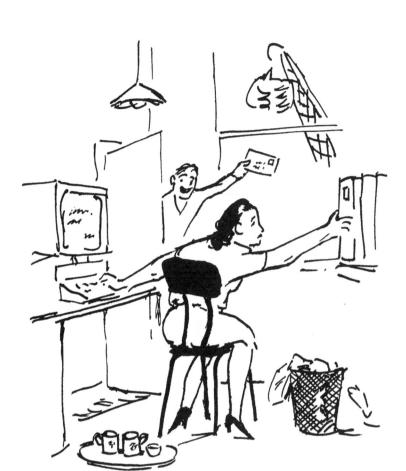

An awkward place to work

---

these extremes, it is at least essential that supervisors are aware of the
potential problems.

Lack of understanding of the potential problem may cause affected
individuals to continue at work which will enormously aggravate and
prolong the problem.

Good Jobs and Bad Jobs

Much has been written about the importance of the position in which people work. Examples are easy to find of workers who have been required to operate an assembly line which is too low, requiring them to stoop forwards or too high, requiring them to maintain elevation of their shoulders which will sooner or later cause trouble. Painting ceilings or working under cars are jobs in which these sort of positions are unavoidable, but in many instances changes in design at the workplace or changes in equipment can solve the problem.

Studies have clearly shown that problems are most likely to arise from a combination of force and repetition and much more likely to occur in women than in men. Thus tasks combining high force and high repetition rates are more likely to cause trouble than those with either high force or high repetition rate; these are in turn more likely to cause trouble than jobs requiring a low force and with a low rate of repetition.

There is much more to a good working environment than the position in which the work is carried out.

A good job has:

✔　　**Variety**

✔　　**Opportunity** - to learn
                  - to innovate

✔　　**Elbow Room** - physical comfort

✔　　**Autonomy**

✔　　**Mental Challenge**

✔　　**Involvement**

✔　　**Colleagues** - nice ones

✔　　**Prospects**

The importance of avoiding repetitive work does not require emphasis. It is not hard to see that workers who have a personal interest in the success of their company and who have the opportunity to develop, to suggest, to rise, will be more likely to perform well and will be more likely to enjoy their work. It is not hard to see that supervision and the monitoring of work rates and output are a serious source of stress. Thus autonomy is preferable to a system in which all must work to the same targets, the same for every minute of every day. People are not the same and one person is not the same at all times. It is not only RSI but several other medical problems which have been found to occur more frequently in those who have no control over their jobs, for example people working on a production line. Attitudes of other workers, in particular managers, are also relevant. We cannot expect to choose our workmates and even if we did, we would probably make the same mistakes which we make with marriages! What is needed is a little luck, a great deal of patience and a lot of hard work to maintain relationships.

The Secretarial Position

RSI is epidemic because of keyboard workers and because there are so many of them. If it had been restricted to chicken pluckers, this book would never have been written. Keyboard workers therefore deserve special emphasis and their work station is undoubtedly important. The ideal work station is illustrated (page 56). Since secretaries and other types of keyboard workers are not all the same size, the equipment, the height of the chair and the back support in particular, must be adjustable. The secretary must be able to sit with her feet touching the floor, with her forearms horizontal at the level of the keyboard so that her wrists are at or near the neutral position. If its a "him", the same considerations apply. The distance from eyes to screen must be comfortable and a document holder if required, must be at the same distance. Neither the screen nor the document holder may be placed at the side of the desk as this would require the head to be turned while working. Screen and eyes must be at about the same height. There must be adequate leg room and a comfortable back support.

Rules for Keyboard Workers

Apart from work stations, there are important rules for secretaries and airline reservation clerks, journalists and other keyboard workers, the general principles of which apply to all workers.

- **Get Fit** before you go to work. Marathon runners and javelin throwers don't go out to pursue their tasks without extensive preparation and work is the same. Regular healthy exercise in people who do physical work is essential. It is madness to go out and run a marathon without preparation; it is equally madness to turn up at an office and type all day without any preparation. An eye check is essential for all screen users.

- **Don't Type All Day** - it causes RSI. Job rotation is the ideal solution, some typing some filing, some telephone work. Recommendations about the maximum amount of keyboard work vary. It is said that in Australia, few women spend more than fifty percent of their day on a keyboard but this is an extreme view – Seventy five percent would be a reasonable target.

- **Take Regular Breaks** - again opinions vary about the times but for intensive keyboard work, fifteen minutes every hour is recommended and for ordinary keyboard work, fifteen minutes every two hours. Job rotation is a more efficient solution.

- **Change Position Regularly**

- **Beware of Stress** - yes, beware of deadlines, demanding bosses (the stick) and bonuses and incentives (the carrot).

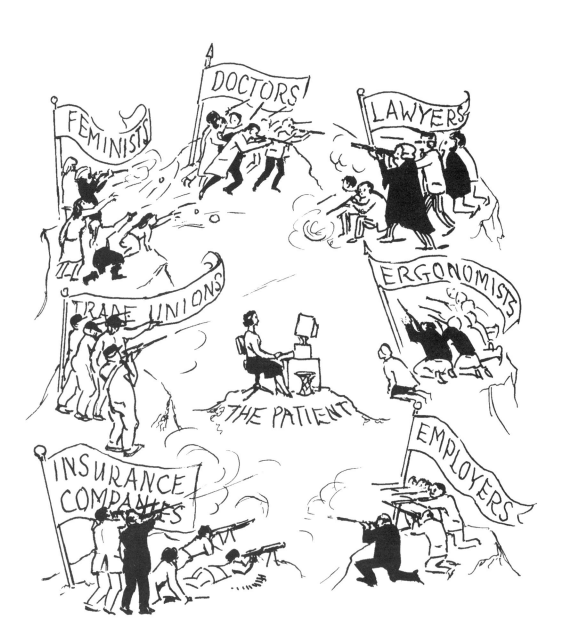

The battle of RSI

CHAPTER 9

Legal Aspects and Compensation

RSI has hit the headlines with a few large and several small awards to sufferers. Potential litigants should however be warned that they are unlikely to be successful, that they are unlikely to get much money and that the process is likely to be long and unpleasant. It may delay their recovery and is best avoided. Their chances of obtaining compensation for an industrial injury from the Department of Social Security are even more bleak.

The Employers Duty

The employers responsibilities can be summarised as follows:

✔ To provide a safe place of work

✔ To avoid exposure of employees to unnecessary risks including repetitive work, or prolonged work in the same position without adequate breaks or variety of tasks

✔ To provide competent fellow employees

✔ To provide adequate supervision at work

✔ To maintain plant and facilities

✔ To provide adequate training and safe systems at work

✔ To warn of any particular hazards

✔ To heed the employees complaints and take appropriate action

These duties are based on the following:

● The Factories Act 1961

● The Offices Shops and Railway Premises Act 1963

● Employers Liability (defective equipment) 1969

● Health and Safety at Work 1974

● EEC Council Directive of 29th May 1990 reported in the official Journal of the European Communities of 21/6/90.

● Health and Safety Information Bulletin 176, August 1990

● HSC draft regulations of 23/1/92

● Case Law

The EEC directive is particularly important for keyboard workers and it is very specific in its requirements. It becomes legally enforceable for work stations put into service after the last day of 1992 and employers must take steps to ensure that work stations put into service prior to this date are adapted within four years - plenty of time! Article seven is worthy of reproduction.

DAILY WORK ROUTINE

The employer must plan the workers activities in such a way that daily work on a display screen is periodically interrupted by breaks or changes of activity, reducing the workload at the display screen.

The annex provides the detailed minimum requirements of the keyboard, work surface and chair as well as the environment, space, heating, lighting, noise and humidity.

How to Succeed with a Claim

Three things must be established by the plaintiff:

● injury

● that the injury is work related

● fault or negligence

In order to make a successful claim it is necessary to establish that an injury has occurred, that it is work related and that the employer failed in some aspect of his duty of care to the employee. It has been surprisingly easy to establish the presence of injury in RSI, especially considering that there is usually nothing objective to find, no swellings, missing limbs or deformities. In some cases, there have been surgical scars, although it is now clear that such surgery was inappropriate and unsuccessful. There are no X-Ray changes and there is no other hard evidence - just the patient's description of the pain.

The employer may fail to defend the case if he has set tasks requiring repetitive movements or prolonged work in the same position without adequate breaks or variation of tasks, insisted on a strict production schedule, provided an unsatisfactory work station, failed to provide adequate training, or to warn of potential risks or to listen to complaints when they were made. However time is of the essence – be quick – there is a three year time limit for accident and injury claims. Remember that your lawyer needs time to prepare your case.

The Duty to Warn

Failure to provide an adequate warning to employees has been a feature of several successful suits. The matter is extensively argued in the case of Presland v Padley. The plaintiff (Presland) in this case was employed in a factory processing chickens. She passed a dexterity test and after a training period was then employed either trussing or weighing chickens. Her thumbs, hands and arms started to ache from the time she started work and as is so characteristic of RSI, she recovered in the evenings. After a few months at work, her right forearm became swollen and a diagnosis of tenosynovitis was made. She made two allegations of negligence, that she was made to work too fast, and that she was not given a specific warning of the risk of tenosynovitis. On the first count, the judge did not accept her allegation but on the second she was successful. Examination of the first aid book at her place of work revealed eighteen cases of tenosynovitis in as many months and in the same period there were one hundred and sixty eight cases of strain to the thumbs, hands and wrists. The defendants, the employers, knew of the risk; the plaintiff did not. It was their duty to tell her of the risk. In judge speak, "an employer is under a duty in cases where the work causes an inherent, specific and not insignificant risk of a servant developing an industrial disease or condition to tell the servant at the beginning of the employment about the risk in order to allow the servant the option whether to embark on the employment or not." In this case, the nurse at the work place suggested, not unreasonably, that if employees were warned, they might have the idea that they had the condition when they had not - auto-suggestion, she called it. If employees knew of the risk, they might not work quite so happily. But the judge was not impressed. Nor was he impressed by the patient's failure to get better. At the end of the trial she continued to complain of pain in her hands but the judge found that a causal connection between this pain and her work had not been established. The plaintiff was awarded £1,250, now equivalent to about twice that sum together with costs and interest. Reading the case, there is surely no doubt that she had RSI although she may also have had tenosynovitis.

Not only must an employer warn of risk, but he (or she) must document the warnings. An unrecorded warning is of no value in law. Furthermore there must be a process of continuing education, also documented, to maintain the employee's awareness of the risks to which he or she is exposed.

The Need to Heed

An employee of the Midland Bank in Nottingham was awarded £45,000 in an out of court settlement for "tenosynovitis". She was a secretary. Her pain started when she moved from a low desk to a higher one; her wrists became painful and two operations failed to solve the problem. A very important aspect of the case was the attitude of her manager who repeatedly ignored her complaints of searing pain in her arms, wrists and hands and her requests for a new work station. Employers and their representatives who manage or supervise those doing manual work must now be aware of this potential problem and be able to take appropriate steps if it arises.

Diagnostic Problems

There is considerable confusion about the exact diagnosis in many of the successful RSI cases; the disease is variously called carpal tunnel syndrome, tenosynovitis or tennis elbow. In one case there was also osteoarthritis, a much more serious condition which could not be expected to resolve. The Daily Telegraph (28/4/92) reported "record damages for strain injury" awarded to a former Vauxhall machine operator. She spent two years loading up to five hundred gear wheels a day, a job requiring force, turning and twisting. Although she started with aching in her fingers, she went on to develop osteoarthritis in her left thumb and parts of her hand. She was awarded £59,617 in damages, made up of £12,000 for the injury itself, £31,454 for loss of earnings, £1,000 for being handicapped on the job market and interest. She expected £7,000 and was reported to be planning a months holiday in St Lucia to celebrate!

Quantum – How Much?

The level of damages which a successful claim for RSI will produce usually lies between £2,000 and £6,000. In addition, it should be possible to recover lost earnings, expenses such as medical bills and the legal costs. In line with this, nine employees of Letraset shared £19,000 in 1991 for various upper limb disorders including tenosynovitis, carpal tunnel syndrome, tennis elbow and trigger thumb. Two employees at British Telecom were awarded £6,000 each for tennis elbow. Unsuccessful surgery seems to increase the level of the award which will also depend on age, employment prospects, loss of earnings and the severity and duration of symptoms.

Who Pays?

Lawyers are expensive; a day in court costs about £6,000 and up to that stage, every letter and medical report must be paid for. The union may help and legal aid is also a possibility

Social Security

An employee who is unable to work because of RSI will receive statutory sick pay. A medical certificate is required.

RSI is not covered by the industrial injuries disablement benefit scheme, set out in leaflets NI2 and NI6 from the Department of Health and Social Security. There are various types of accepted industrial injury; the two closest to RSI are cramps and tenosynovitis.

Cramps are a very rare source of benefit but tenosynovitis accounts for up to one third of all prescribed diseases.

Disease No	Name of Disease Or Injury	Type of Job
A4	Cramp of the hand or forearm due to repetitve movements. For example, writer's cramp.	Prolonged periods of handwriting, typing or other repetitive movements of the finger, hand or arm. For example, typists, clerks and routine assemblers.
A8	Traumatic inflammation of the tendons of the hand or forearm, or of the associated tendon sheaths.	Manual labour, or frequent or repeated movements of the hand or wrist. For example, routine assembly workers.

How to Claim

- Fill in form B1 100 B (get it from the DHSS) within three months of being entitled.

- Expect some delay, then enquiries from an adjudication officer, perhaps followed by a referral to a specialist and attendance at a medical board which will make a decision about eligibility and the degree of disability. Appeals can be made at all stages.

What Will Happen

Probably nothing. Benefit is only paid when the degree of disability is assessed at over 14%. In RSI, it is usually less. This scheme is for exciting injuries like the loss of an arm or a leg. Loss of both hands is assessed at 100% but they must be cut off - not rendered useless by a disease like RSI. Loss of an index finger is assessed at 14%.

Industrial Tribunal

An employee may also seek redress from an industrial tribunal for wrongful dismissal and loss of earnings.

CHAPTER 10

Prevention, Management and Outcome

Prevention is the most important and most successful strategy for RSI. The failure of various treatments, the so-called refractory nature of the condition, has already been noted as one of it's major characteristics.

Prevention

There are two aspects of prevention. Primary prevention means stopping the condition from arising and is the best that can be achieved. There is no doubt that a radical change will have to occur in the attitudes of employers to allow careful examination of the workplace of all employees and their work plans. Many many secretaries and other keyboard workers spend all day on a machine and this cannot continue. Secondary prevention means the prompt recognition of the condition so that measures can be taken to minimise it's consequences. In the early case, a short rest followed by a return to a modified work regime with improvements in the use of equipment if necessary will often avert the disaster of full-blown RSI. The design of the workplace and optimal conditions of work are discussed in chapter 8.

Management

It is unfortunate that there have been few scientifically acceptable studies of the effects of treatment in RSI. There has been only one reported study in which groups of patients were treated in different ways so that the results could be compared. This is a trial of cognitive-behavioural therapy which is discussed in detail below. There is no study comparing an anti-inflammatory drug and placebo; we know that placebo, dummy tablets or injections or almost anything else, will have a beneficial effect in some patients even if their problems are due to something quite serious like rheumatoid arthritis. Most recommendations on treatment must therefore be based on experience. And experience is notoriously fallacious. There is an urgent need for proper studies.

Careful and Compassionate Explanation • Reassurance • Advice

Many patients with RSI complain that their problem was not at first recognised. The absence of physical signs may encourage the view that there is nothing wrong although patients with angina no longer have difficulty in persuading their doctors to accept their story of pain recurring on exercise even though their hearts sound normal through the stethoscope. The search for relief and belief - for recognition as genuinely sick - has been described as a pilgrimage of pain. The very least that a patient can expect is therefore a reasonable explanation of the problem together with a plan for the future and some idea of what will happen next.

The occupation of the patient is central to the advice which will be given. This, together with the likely outcome, is discussed in greater detail below.

Rest and Exercise

Rest is the first essential in the management of RSI and is the only certain way of relieving the pain. Patients who develop RSI while carrying out a particular task must be removed from that task and allowed to rest until the pain has resolved.

It may seem contradictory but there is a strong impression that exercise and physical fitness are helpful in the management of RSI. This approach is certainly central to the management of the closely related condition fibromyalgia. In this condition, a graduated (slowly increasing) programme of muscle-building exercise is used to relieve

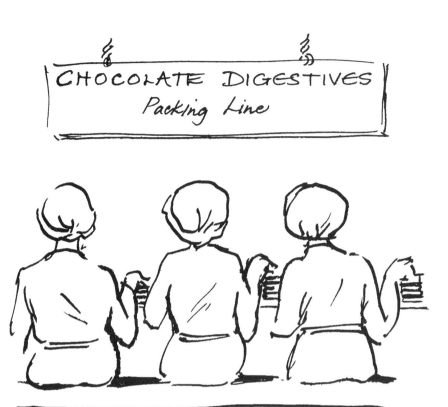

A change of

the pain and in the long term, to prevent recurrence. Because warmth relieves the pain and buoyancy in water makes it easier to move stiff limbs, hydrotherapy is often used to initiate treatment. Exercise is used in the management of other chronic pain syndromes. Some argue that it is the release of endorphins, the body's natural pain-relieving and euphoria-inducing opiates, which explains the efficacy of exercise. It is common sense to expect that a chronic pain sufferer

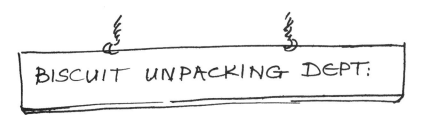

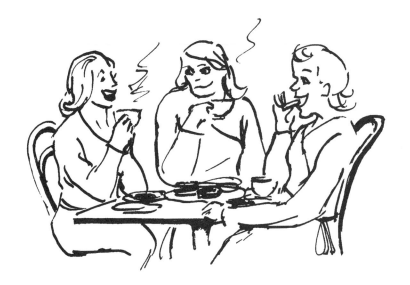

occupation

who is exercising regularly and has become physically fit will be happier than another who spends all day in front of the television doing nothing. A graduated exercise programme designed to achieve aerobic fitness is a useful part of the programme of treatment of RSI and when the time to return to work comes, the fitter patient has a better chance of avoiding a recurrence of symptoms.

Early Return to Work • Alternative Employment

Most authorities agree that an early return to work is the best plan in RSI and that the longer a return to work is delayed, the more difficult it becomes. Some have suggested that patients should go to their workplace even if they cannot take any part in their usual job. By the time the patient returns to work, modifications must have been made to prevent recurrence of symptoms. It is obvious that if a patient returns to exactly the same work which caused the problem, the symptoms will recur and experience confirms that this is so. The return to work must be guided, supported and supervised.

In severe cases, it may be impossible to return to keyboard or other manual work and recovery may take years. In these circumstances it may be necessary to advise a change of occupation. It is surprising how many occupations, especially those carried out by women, require repetitive manual work. There are however a few things which one might consider:

Possible occupations for women with RSI who cannot return to their usual occupations

- Receptionist
- Traffic Warden
- Shop Worker
- Interpreter
- Charity Worker
- Adviser/information officer
- Broadcaster
- Actress
- Sales representative
- Politician

- Counsellor
- Social Worker
- Teacher
- Buyer
- Audiovisual technician
- Customs officer
- Estate agent
- Dietician
- Market researcher
- Personnel officer

Counselling and Cognitive-Behavioural Therapy

Cognitive-behavioural therapy has been tested in a unique controlled trial, the only one in RSI, and found to be effective. In the study, patients were allocated to three groups at random. One remained on a waiting list while the others were treated either by an individual therapist or in a group. One might make one small criticism of this design because the waiting list group had absolutely no treatment. Almost anything which is done to patients will be better than nothing at all! In other studies of this type, the problem has been overcome by seeing all patients at the same intervals. The untreated patients could have had a cup of tea with an untrained person who would have provided a better comparison to the psychotherapists. Nevertheless, the results of the study were very straightforward and very convincing.

Not surprisingly, patients kept on a waiting list for treatment remained exactly the same or were slightly worse over a two month period. In the same period, there were striking improvements in the treated groups. Their pain improved, they became less depressed and less anxious and their pain had less effect on their ability to carry out everyday tasks, such as looking after themselves and their ability to get on with other people and to function in the community. In other words, their RSI had less impact on their lives. Patients treated individually did a little better than those treated in a group and after the end of the treatment, they tended to continue to improve whereas in some respects, the patients treated in groups deteriorated. Treatment did not seem to increase the likelihood of a return to work although treated patients tended to require less medication. The biggest effect of the treatment was to enable patients to "cope" with their pain even though it was still present.

What is cognitive-behavioural therapy and what is involved? Patients in the study had nine sessions with a psychotherapist each lasting for an hour and a half. They had homework between sessions. The components of the treatment were:

- **goal setting**, for example encouraging patients to increase their activities, to re-establish broken relationships with their friends and perhaps workmates, and to increase reinforcing events and activities

- **cognitive restructuring**, which means sorting out patients' ideas about their condition and their pain, correcting false beliefs and accepting that depression and anxiety may play a part in maintaining chronic pain

- **relaxation training**, teaching patients to break the pain-tension-pain cycle, to relax instead of tensing up during stressful or repetitive activities

- **learning skills for coping with pain**, for example using images or distraction to get away from pain

- **correcting sleep disturbances** with relaxation techniques, sophisticated psychological developments of the old method of counting sheep

- **training in communication and assertion skills**; teaching female secretaries to refuse to accept an unreasonable pile of work from an aggressive male manager without causing too much trouble, to be able to ask for changes in equipment and to manage their working time in a better way

Some doctors would argue that counselling is part of their role in looking after their patients but for those who don't have time or prefer to use the skills of trained therapists, referral to a counsellor seems a good idea in RSI. The counsellor elicits the patients problems and losses, the anger and frustration and the depression. Identification and exploration of these problems may lead to solutions and also to a recognition of what is left and what can be done with it, a positive approach in place of a negative one.

Sleep

Disturbed sleep adds to the problem of pain as it does in fibromyalgia. Loss of the deep refreshing bits of sleep (delta sleep) makes muscles tense, tight and uncomfortable even in healthy people. If the muscles are already painful as in RSI, the situation is worse. Breaking the vicious cycle of disturbed sleep and muscle pain is an essential part of treatment. If counting sheep doesn't work, a small dose of amitriptylene (10mg increased if necessary) at night may be a good idea and is certainly harmless. It is wise to avoid benzodiazepines like diazepam which are habit-forming.

Physiotherapy

Physiotherapists can do lots of things. They are not however trained as psychotherapists although many are skillful at talking to patients at the same time as treating them. Referral to a physiotherapist should therefore be for a specific purpose, with a well defined plan and with regular assessment of progress.

Things that physiotherapists do - and might be asked to do for patients with RSI.

- Mobilisation of stiff bits

- Immobilization of mobile bits

- Heat and cold

- Massage and friction

- Correction of posture

- Electrotherapy (ultrasound etc)

- Exercise programmes

- Relaxation techniques

- Acupuncture and acupressure

- Adverse mechanical tension techniques

Most of these techniques are spectacularly unsuccessful in RSI, as are most other forms of treatment. The value of an exercise programme has already been discussed. It is possible to achieve transient relief of pain with things like heat or cold or at greater cost with electrical machines but it is unlikely that this influences the course of the condition. On the other hand, patients with RSI need someone to talk to and why not a physiotherapist? Or does attending a physiotherapist for months of unsuccessful treatment encourage a client to retain the sick role? It's a dilemma which must be considered for each individual patient. Most of the treatments listed overleaf will usually fail. Some will help a bit and very very slowly, most patients actually get better. None of these techniques is of proven value. None has been tested in any kind of study. Shame!

Splints

Wrist splints seem to help in some cases. As with collars for bad necks, the use of a splint for a short time in the acute stage is entirely acceptable. The use of splints in the long term may perpetuate the problem by adding the hazards of immobilisation to those of repetition. Upon return to work, arm rests fitted to the secretarial chair, may help to support the forearm and wrist.

Things to Avoid

Soft tissue injections don't work in RSI although they may give transient relief of pain. The problem is not an enthesitis or a tensynovitis and injecting the muscle insertion or tendon sheath won't solve it. Surgery is a disaster, unnecessary, unsuccessful and likely to make things worse by adding a scar, a real injury to an already difficult situation. The quest for compensation is also unhelpful and will delay recovery. There is an obvious conflict. On the one hand, the patient is seeing doctors and therapists hoping to get better. On the other, the same patient must convince often sceptical and antagonistic lawyers and doctors acting for employers or their insurers, about their injury, it's severity and it's duration. Patients are sometimes encouraged by unrealistic levels of compensation suggested by trade union representatives or fellow employees. But they should be warned that the quest for compensation will be long, slow and unpleasant. The outcome will probably be disappointing except for the lawyers who always win! Drugs are not the answer and there is nothing in the health food shop which solves the problem.

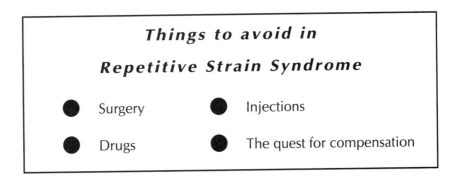

Things to avoid in

Repetitive Strain Syndrome

- Surgery
- Injections
- Drugs
- The quest for compensation

Outcome

RSI almost always gets better with time and rest, care and a little kindness. There are many figures in the literature, varying widely and presumably depending on the severity of the cases. A specialist referral centre will see only the worst cases while an occupational physician in a well-run company will see many which are trivial. A Japanese study representing the middle of the road and conforming to my own experience found a mean recovery time of 4.6 years in cash register operatives. Within three years 36% had recovered, within five 64% and within ten 94%. The moral is repeated again and again...

● **prevent it if possible but if it happens, recognise it quickly and take appropriate action.**

Appendix 1

References and suggestions for further reading

History

Quintner J 1991

The RSI syndrome in historical perspective.

International Disability Studies, 13, 99-104.

The Cause

Cohen ML, Arroyo JF, Champion GD and Browne CD 1992

In search of the pathogenesis of refractory cervicobrachial pain syndrome.

The Medical Journal of Australia 156, 432-6.

The Australian epidemic

Bell DS 1989

"Repetition strain injury": an iatrogenic epidemic of simulated injury.

The Medical Journal of Australia 151, 280-4.

Meekosha H and Jakubowicz A 1991

Repetition strain injury: The rise and fall of an "Australian" disease.

Critical Social Policy 11, 18-37.

Ferguson DA 1987

"RSI": putting the epidemic to rest.

The Medical Journal of Australia, 147, 213-4.

U.S. experience

Hadler NM 1992

Arm pain in the workplace. A small area analysis.

Journal of Occupational Medicine, 34,113-9.

The orthodox orthopaedic viewpoint

(RSI doesn't exist!)

Campbell Semple J 1991

Tenosynovitis, repetitive strain injury, cumulative trauma disorder, and overuse syndrome, et cetera.

Journal of Bone and Joint Surgery (British edition) 73 B, 536-8.

Diagnosis and treatment

Browne CD, Nolan BM and Faithfull DK 1984

Occupational repetition strain injuries. Guidelines for diagnosis and management.

The Medical Journal of Australia 140, 329-32.

The controlled trial of cognitive behavioural therapy

Spence SH 1989

Cognitive-behaviour therapy in the management of chronic occupational pain of the upper limbs.

Behaviour Research of Therapy, 27, 435-46.

Chicken process workers and their problems

Buckle P 1987

Musculoskeletal disorders of the upper extremities: The use of epidemiologic approaches in industrial settings.

The Journal of Hand Surgery, 12 A, 885-9.

Musicians and their problems

Fry HJH 1986

Overuse syndrome of the upper limb in musicians.

The Medical Journal of Australia, 144, 182-5.

Appendix 2

Where to get help if you have RSI.

RSI Association,

Clone House,

Highbridge Estate,

Oxford Road,

Uxbridge,

Middlesex UB8 1UL.

Telephone 0895 238663.

Charterhouse Health Series

Forthcoming titles:

- Complimentary Medicine

- Smoking

- Exercise Medicine

- Heart Attacks and Strokes

"Books for doctors that patients can read...

...Books for patients that doctors can read"

Published by
Charterhouse Conference and Communications Limited
35 Cloth Fair, London EC1A 7JQ.
Tel: 071-606 2435. Fax: 071-606 2351